Maissa Ben Thayer
Fatma Khanchel
Imen Helal

Ki67 in breast carcinoma

Maissa Ben Thayer
Fatma Khanchel
Imen Helal

Ki67 in breast carcinoma

Correlation with prognostic factors

ScienciaScripts

Imprint

Any brand names and product names mentioned in this book are subject to trademark, brand or patent protection and are trademarks or registered trademarks of their respective holders. The use of brand names, product names, common names, trade names, product descriptions etc. even without a particular marking in this work is in no way to be construed to mean that such names may be regarded as unrestricted in respect of trademark and brand protection legislation and could thus be used by anyone.

Cover image: www.ingimage.com

This book is a translation from the original published under ISBN 978-620-3-44168-0.

Publisher:
Sciencia Scripts
is a trademark of
Dodo Books Indian Ocean Ltd. and OmniScriptum S.R.L Publishing group
Str. Armeneasca 28/1, office 1, Chisinau-2012, Republic of Moldova, Europe
Printed at: see last page
ISBN: 978-620-5-26654-0

BEN THAYER MAISSA KHANCHEL FATMA

HELAL IMEN

KI67 IN BREAST CARCINOMA: CORRELATION WITH MAJOR

FACTORS

PROGNOSIS

OCTOBER 2022

TABLE OF CONTENTS

INTRODUCTION

Breast carcinoma (BC) is the most common cancer of all types worldwide and the fourth leading cause of cancer death worldwide, with more than 2.2 million new cases diagnosed and 650,000 deaths in 2020 [1].

In Tunisia, the incidence of SC has increased steadily over the past twenty years and is still promoted to rise with a standardized incidence rate expected in 2040 to 122.5/100000 inhabitants [2]. SC is the most frequent cancer in our country, representing in 2021, 15.9% of all newly diagnosed cancers. It is the second leading cause of cancer mortality [1].

The CS, thus constitutes, because of its frequency and its gravity, a true problem of public health in Tunisia.Despite the efforts made in terms of screening and the progress of the therapeutic arsenal, the prognosis of CS remains rather reserved. The mortality rate of CS in women of reproductive age in Tunisia reaches 33.02% [3].

The role of the pathologist is essential, not only in the diagnosis of SC but also in the determination of histopronostic factors essential to the adequate therapeutic management of patients and to the establishment of the post-therapeutic surveillance strategy.The biology of SC is constantly evolving and is of increasing interest to pathologists around the world. Currently, the therapeutic strategy in SC is based not only on the TNM stage, but also on the molecular classification of the tumor [4].

The main biological markers guiding adjuvant therapy in breast cancer were estrogen receptor (ER), progesterone receptor (PR) and epidermal growth factor (HER2) levels [5].

However, in recent years, many studies have revealed that proliferation markers, and mainly Ki67, are predictive of prognosis of SC but also of response to adjuvant therapy.Ki67, a nuclear antigen of protein nature, is involved in the regulation of the cell cycle and is expressed in all proliferative active phases of this cycle [6]. The Ki67 index, determined by immunohistochemistry, is currently accepted as a marker of tumor proliferation in SC [5].

The prognostic value of Ki67 index in CS has been widely studied. Several studies had established that a high Ki67 index was associated with a worse prognosis, higher mortality and a higher risk of recurrence [4,7].

However, few studies have looked at the correlation of the Ki67 index with other prognostic factors for CS.

The objectives of this work were to :

- To study the clinico-pathological characteristics of CS in a university hospital in northern Tunisia.
- To evaluate the correlation of Ki67 index with the main prognostic factors of CS.

MATERIAL AND METHODS

1. Study Materials:

1.1. Location and time of study:

This was a retrospective descriptive observational study conducted in the Department of Anatomy and Cytology Pathology of Habib Thameur Hospital, Tunis. It concerned cases of breast carcinoma (BC) diagnosed in the department and collected over a five-year period from January 1, 2016 to December 31, 2021.

1.2. Patients:

1.2.1. Inclusion criteria:

We included cases of primary CS diagnosed at the Department of Anatomy and Cytology Pathology of Habib Thameur Hospital during the study period, and having undergone curative surgical treatment.

1.2.2. Non-inclusion criteria:

We did not include in the study: cases of CS :

- histological type other than carcinoma (lymphoma, sarcoma, melanoma, tumor neuroendocrine...).

- diagnosed on biopsies and for which the anatomopathological examination of the corresponding surgical specimen was not performed in our department.

- for which the immunuhistochemical study of the ki67 index was not performed on the surgical specimen.

1.2.3. Exclusion Criteria

Excluded from the study were: cases of CS :

- who received neoadjuvant treatment.

- diagnosed in men

- whose immunuhistochemical study of the ki67 index was non-contributory due to the poor initial fixation of the surgical parts.

2. Methods:

2.1. Collection of clinical, anatomopathological data:

The data were collected on a standardized form, pre-established for each patient, after consultation of the anatomopathological reports obtained from the computerized archiving software of the service, and after examination of the histological sections stored in the archives of the service.

All the data were transcribed in a table of the Excel software version 2010: Age of the patient
Size of the tumor

Histological type according to the WHO classification 2019 5th edition

Histological grade according to the SBR classification modified by Ellis and Elston (Nottingham grade)

Architectural grade Mitotic grade.
Nuclear grade

Presence of vascular emboli Presence of perinatal sheathing
Tumor status T, node status N and metastatic status M according to the pTNM classification of
AJCC/UICC 2017 CS

Estrogen receptor (ER) Progesterone receptor (PR) HER2 score

Ki67 Index

Molecular classification

2.2. Technical step:

2.2.1. Techniques for the preparation of histological sections: [8,9]

a) Fixation:

Upon receipt, the surgical specimens are fixed with 10% formalin for 24 to 48 hours.

b) Macroscopic examination:

Once this time has elapsed, macroscopic examination of the surgical specimen is performed (Figure 1). Samples are taken and placed in cassettes.

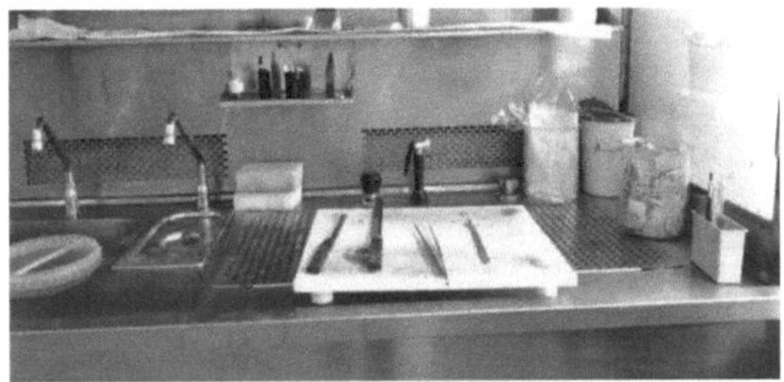

Figure 1 Macroscopic examination table

c) Dehydration:

These cassettes are placed in an inclusion automaton (Figure 2). Thanks to this automaton, the tissue fragments contained in the cassettes will be dehydrated by passing through successive baths of alcohol.

It is necessary to have at least three alcohol baths of increasing concentration 70%, 90% and 100%. This dehydration process is essential to allow the kerosene to penetrate the tissues. The alcohol will be removed by a solvent (mainly xylene).

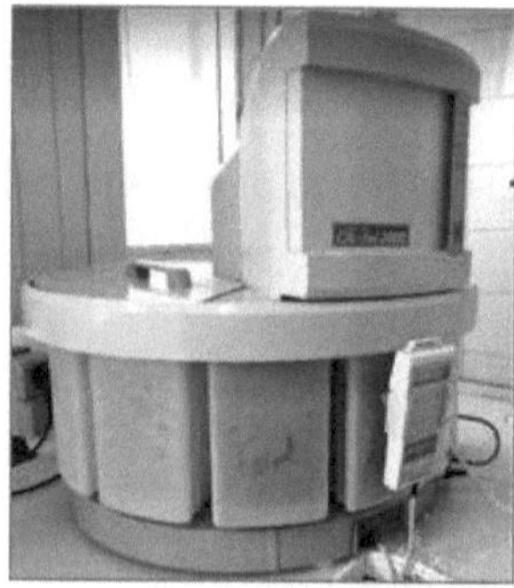

Figure 2 Inclusion automaton

d) Inclusion and molding:

The inclusion medium used is kerosene. Tissue samples are bathed in molten kerosene (heated to 56°C for 4 hours in an oven) which then infiltrates all the cells.After 4 hours of embedding, the liquid kerosene is poured into a small metal mold. After cooling, a hard kerosene block is obtained, inside which the tissue samples are placed.

e) Cup:

After cooling and demolding of the kerosene blocks, 3 to 5 mm thick sections will be made with a microtome (Figure 3). The obtained films are spread on glass slides.

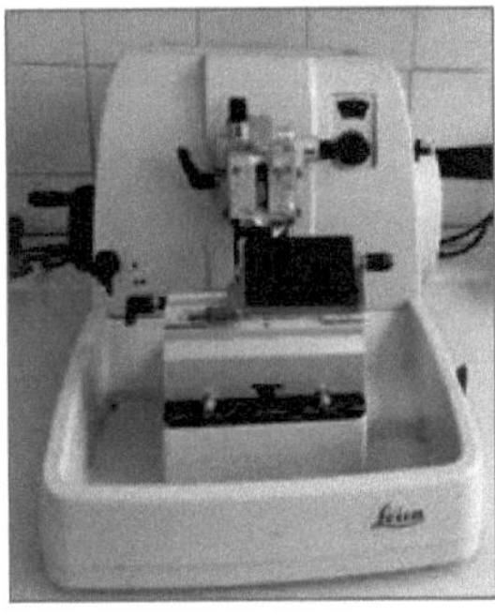

Figure 3 Microtome

f) Dewaxing :

The kerosene is gradually removed by passing the slides through xylene baths.

g) Rehydration:

The slides are placed in alcohol baths of decreasing degrees (from 100° alcohol to 50° alcohol) Figure 4, then in distilled water.

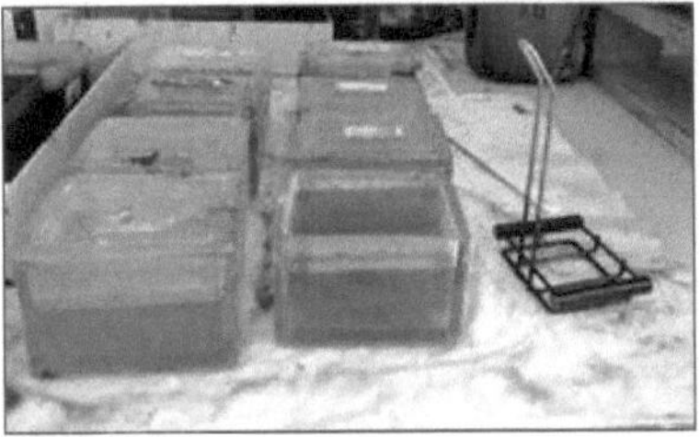

Figure 4 Alcohol baths of decreasing concentration

h) Coloring and editing:

The slides are stained with hemathein-eosin (HE) and a slide-slide mount is performed.

2.2.2. Immunohistochemistry:

Immunohistochemistry consists in highlighting various cellular or extracellular antigens (Ag) using antibodies specifically directed against them, on fixed and paraffin-embedded tissue sections. The revelation of this antigen-antibody complex by a chemical reaction thanks to an enzyme and its substrate [8].

Ki67 index was determined by immunohistochemistry from the preserved kerosene blocks. Sections of 5um were made with a microtome and then placed on slides. Immunohistochemical analyses were performed according to the avidin-biotin complex labelled method using an automaton (the Bond Max) with DAB as chromogen, using a monoclonal antibody, diluted at 1/150.

2.3. Determination of the ki67 index:

To determine the Ki67 score we followed the recommendations of the International Ki67 in Breast Cancer Working Group [10,11] :

• We determined the percentage of infiltrating tumor cells with positive labeling compared with all tumor cells. The count had to be done on at least 500 infiltrating tumor cells.

• Only the nuclear marking was taken into account, regardless of the intensity of this marking (weak, moderate or intense).

• Areas with a dense inflammatory infiltrate, areas with remodeling from the previous biopsy, and areas of necrosis were avoided during counting.

• A complete screening of the slide at low magnification (×100) was performed.

• Subsequently, at least three fields at high magnification (×400) were scanned in order to appreciate the different intensities of marking present on the whole area to be analyzed.

• The counting was done on at least three fields at high magnification (×400). The areas of tumor invasion fronts as well as the Hot Spot areas were counted.

• The threshold for Ki67 assessment was set in our study at 20%.

2.4. Statistical study:

All data was entered using Microsoft Office Excel

Version 2010 and analyzed using SPSS version 25 software.

We performed a descriptive and an analytical study of the series.

2.2.1. Descriptive study:

- Quantitative values were expressed as a mean.

- Qualitative data were expressed as absolute and relative (percentage) frequency.

2.2.2. Analytical study:

The search for an association between the Ki67 index and clinicopathological prognostic factors was analyzed by Chi-square test (for qualitative variables) and Student's T test (for quantitative variables)

The confidence interval (CI) was set at 95% (a p-value of less than 0.05 was statistically significant calculated using a two-tailed test)

1. General presentation of the study population:

We received 84 mastectomy specimens at the Department of Anatomy and Pathological Cytology of Habib Thameur Hospital between January 1, 2016 and December 31, 2021. We excluded 15 cases including 6 cases of patients who had neoadjuvant treatment, eight cases where the Ki67 immunohistochemical study was non-contributory and one case of CS diagnosed in a man. Thus, 69 cases of SC were included in our study. All these cases met the inclusion criteria described above.

Figure 5 summarizes the patient flow.

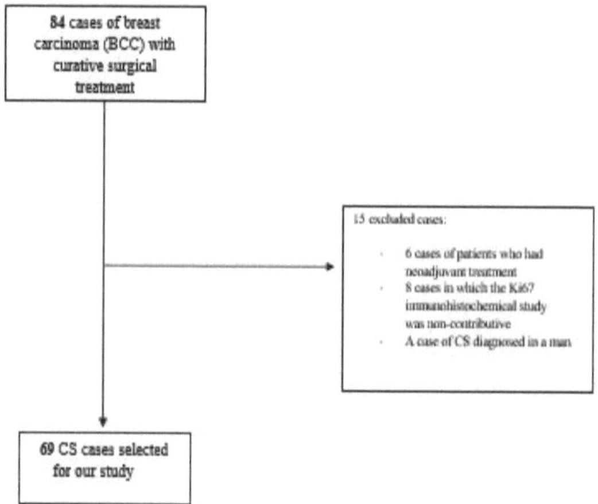

Figure 5 Flow chart: Patient flow by exclusion criteria.

2. Descriptive study:

2.1. Epidemiological characteristics:

2.1.1. Distribution by year of diagnosis:

The 69 cases collected were divided into:

- 12 cases diagnosed in 2016 (17.4% of cases)

- 19 cases diagnosed in 2017 (27.5% of cases)

- 4 cases diagnosed in 2018 (5.7% of cases)

- 15 cases diagnosed in 2019 (21.7% of cases)

- 10 cases diagnosed in 2020 (14.5% of cases)

- 9 cases diagnosed in 2021 (13.2% of cases)

The distribution of cases by year of diagnosis is shown in the Figure 6.

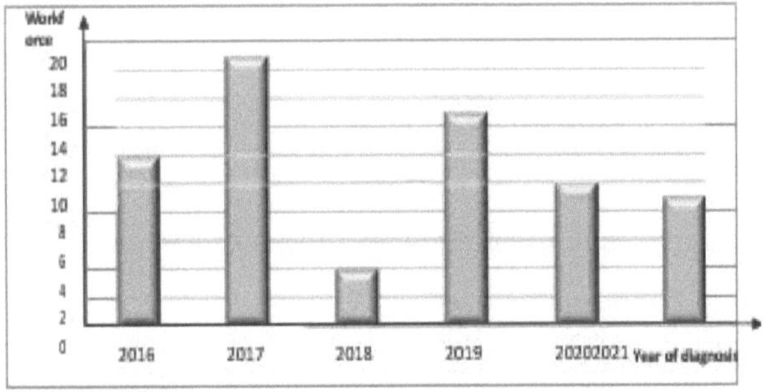

Figure 6 Distribution of cases by year of diagnosis

2.1.2. Age distribution:

The mean age of the patients was 53 ± 13 years with extremes ranging from 23 to 79 years. The peak frequency was between 60-70 years (30.4%) as shown in **Figure 7**.

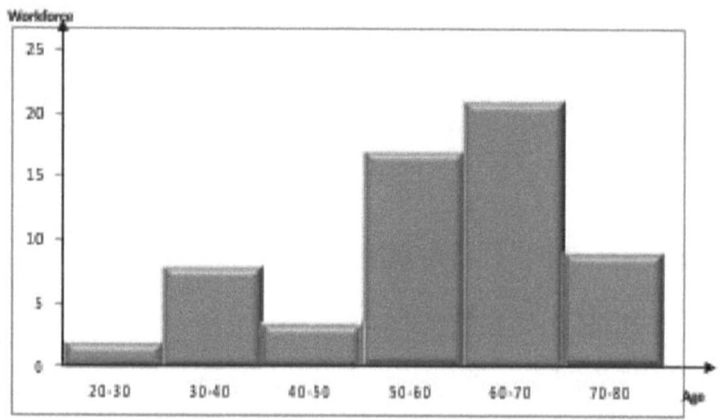

Figure 7 Age distribution of the 69 cases studied

2.2. Pathological characteristics of the tumor:

2.2.1. Distribution by tumor size: Figure 8

Tumor size ranged from 6 to 80mm with a mean of 35.3mm ± 19.3. Cases were subdivided according to tumor size:

- Tumor size ≤ 2 cm (13 cases, 18.8%)
- Tumor size > 2 cm (56 cases, 81.2%)

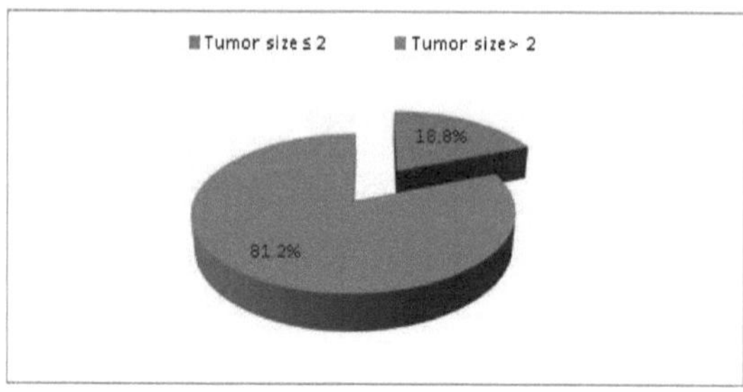

Figure 8 Distribution of tumors by size

2.2.2. Distribution by histological type:

The 69 carcinomas collected were divided into;

- Invasive carcinoma without other indication (NOS), formerly called invasive ductal carcinoma, in 50 cases (72.5%).
- Invasive lobular carcinoma in 11 cases (15.9%).
- Mixed carcinoma six cases (8.7%)
- Micropapillary carcinoma in two cases (2.9%).

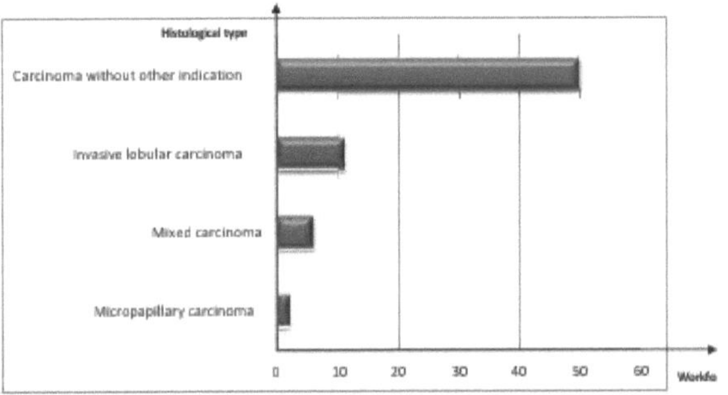

Figure 9 Distribution of tumors according to histological type

2.2.3. Distribution by SBR grade:

In our series :

- 14.5% of the carcinomas were SBR grade I
- 47.8% of the carcinomas were SBR grade II
- 37.7% of the carcinomas were SBR grade II

The distribution of tumors according to SBR grade is shown in Figure 10

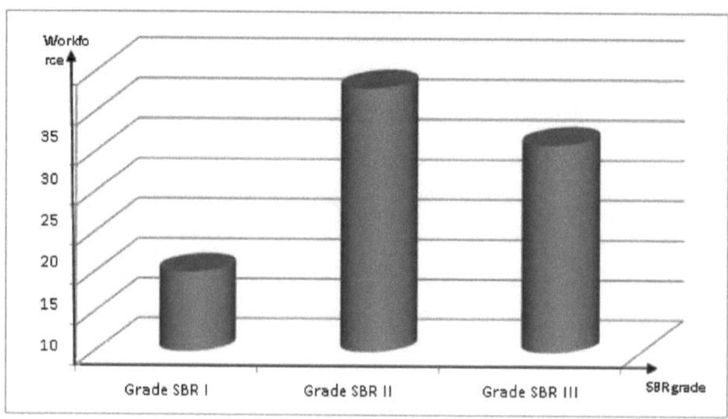

Figure 10 Distribution of tumors according to SBR grade

2.2.4. Distribution according to architectural grade, nuclear grade and mitotic grade:

The distribution of cases according to these three parameters is represented in the Table I:

Table I Distribution of tumors by architectural grade, nuclear grade, and mitotic grade

	Score 1		Score 2		Score 3	
	Number of cases	Percentage	Number of cases	Percentage	Number of cases	Percentage
Architectural grade	10	14,5%	13	18,8%	46	66,7%
Nuclear grade	11	15,9%	32	46,4%	26	37,7%
Grade mitotic	30	43,5%	17	24,6%	22	31,9%

2.2.5. Distribution by pT stage:

In our series, the carcinomas were of stage:

- pT1 in 13% of cases.

- pT2 in 66.7% of cases.

- pT3 in 15.9% of cases.

- pT4 in 4.4% of cases.

The distribution of cases according to pT stage is shown in Figure 11
Distribution of tumors according to pT stage.

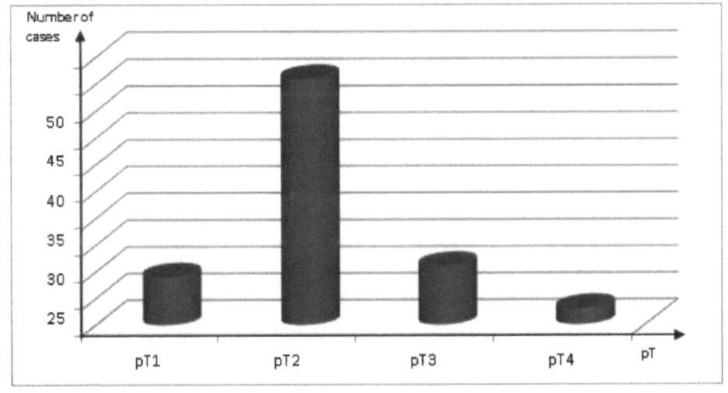

Figure 11 Distribution of tumors according to pT stage

2.2.6. Distribution according to the pN stage:

Lymph node metastases were present in 42 cases (60.8% of cases). The distribution of cases by pN stage is shown in Figure 12.

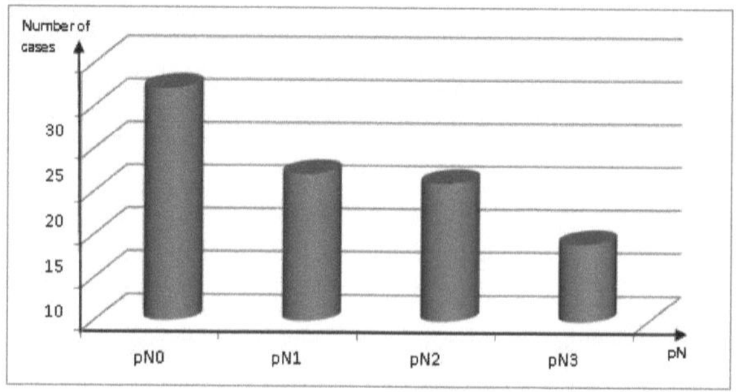

Figure 12 Distribution of tumors by pN stage

2.2.7. Distribution according to the presence of vascular emboli:

Vascular emboli were present in 30.4% of cases (21 cases).

2.2.8. Distribution according to the presence of perineural sheathing:

Perineural sheathing was present in 24.6% of cases (17 cases).

2.2.9. Distribution by estrogen receptor (ER) expression level by tumor cells:

The level of estrogen receptor (ER) expression by tumor cells was :

- ER < 10% in 47 cases (72.4%)

- ER $\geq$ 10% in 22 cases (27.6%)

2.2.10. Distribution according to the level of expression of progesterone receptors (PR) by tumor cells:

The level of progesterone receptor (PR) expression by tumor cells was :

- PR < 10% in 50 cases (68.1%)
- PR ≥ 10% in 19 cases (31.9%)

The distribution of tumors according to ER and PR is shown in Figure 13.

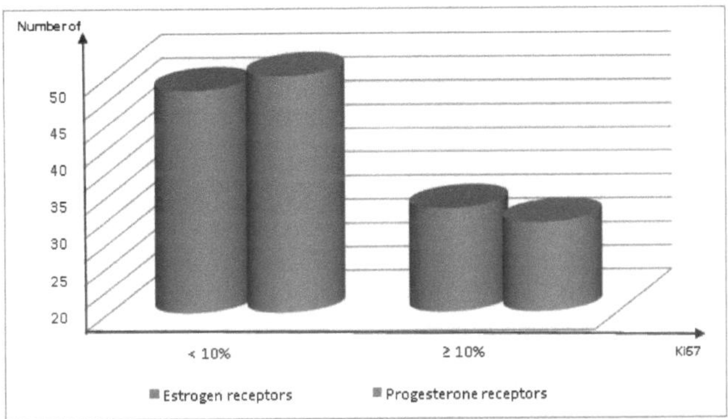

Figure 13 Distribution of tumors according to estrogen receptor (ER) and progesterone receptor (PR)

2.2.11. Distribution by ki67 index: Figure 14

The ki67 index was:

- <20% in 29 cases (42%). Figure 16
- ≥ 20% in 40 cases (58%). Figure 15

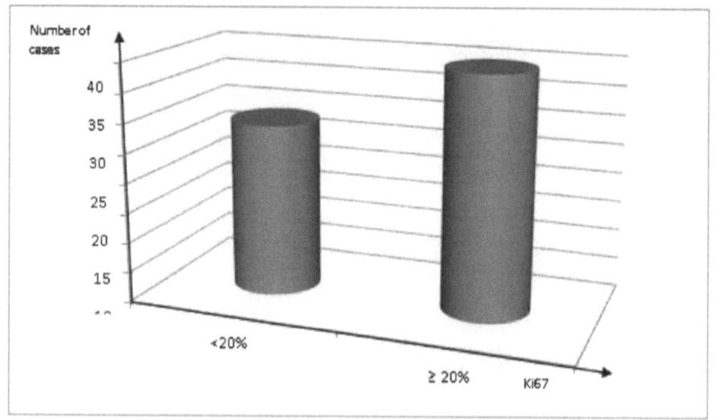

Figure 14 Distribution of tumors according to Ki67

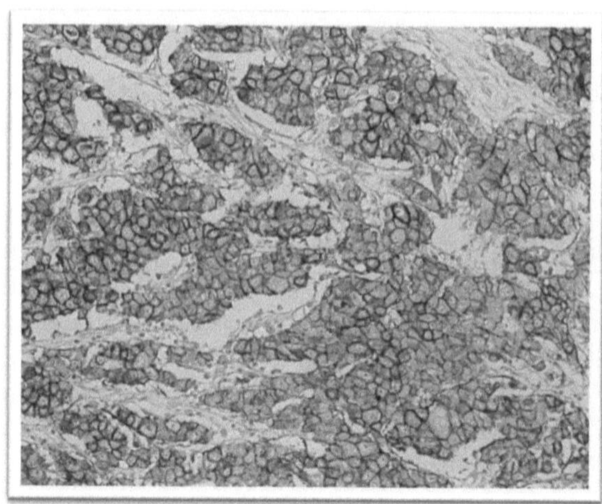

Figure 15 Immunohitochemical study of the Ki67 index: high Ki67 evaluated at 100%.

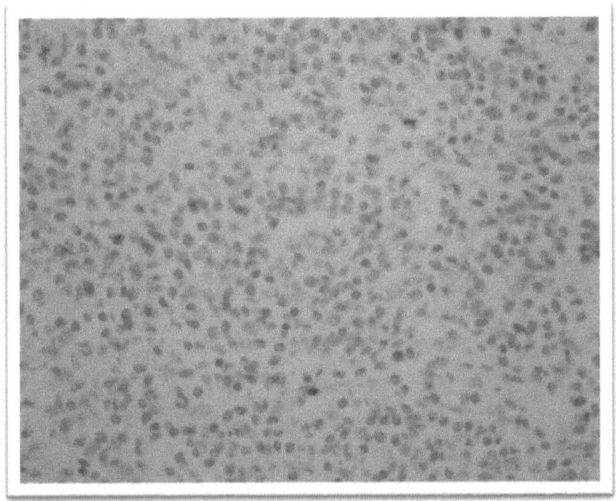

Figure 16 Immunohitochemical study of the Ki67 index: low Ki67 evaluated at 4%.

2.2.12. Distribution by Her2 status:

Her2 was overexpressed in 22 cases (31.9%) and not overexpressed in 47 cases (68.1%).

2.2.13. Distribution according to molecular classification: Figure 17

The 69 cases studied were divided into:

- 20 cases of Luminal class A (29% of cases)
- 33 cases of Luminal B class (47.8% of cases)
- 8 cases of HER2 class (11.6% of cases)
- 8 triple negative cases (11.6% of cases)

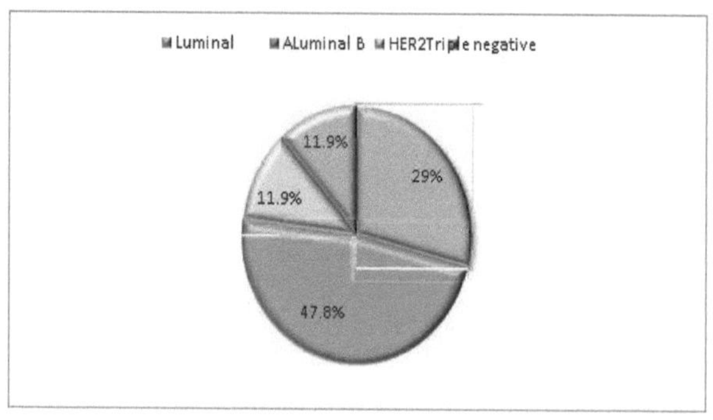

Figure 17 Distribution of tumors according to molecular classification

3. Analytical study:

3.1. Univariate study:

3.1.1. Correlation of Ki67 with age: Figure 18

- Among the 28 patients aged ≤50 years, 14 patients (50% of cases) had a Ki67≥20%.

- Among the 38 patients over 50 years of age, 24 patients (63.1% of cases) had a Ki67≥ 20%.

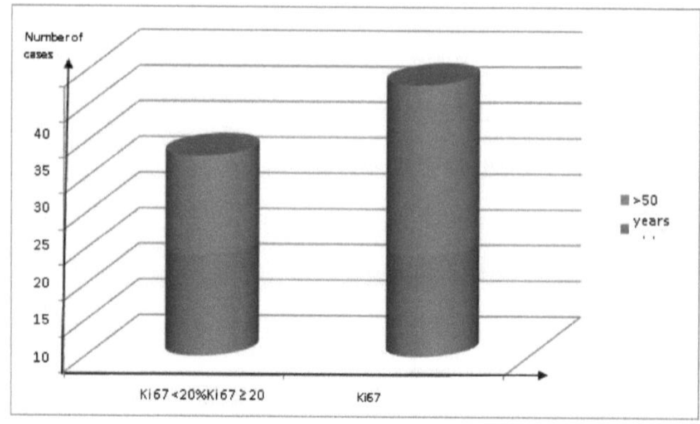

Figure 18 Ki67 index as a function of age

We did not find a statistically significant correlation between Ki67 and age >50 years (p=0.3).By performing the Student's t-test we did not find a statistical correlation between Ki67 and age (p=0.5).

3.1.2. Correlation of Ki67 with height: Figure 19

Of the 29 cases with Ki67 <20%, 24 had a size >2 cm.

Among the 40 cases with Ki67 ≥ 20%, 35 had a size > 2 cm.

We did not find a statistically significant correlation between Ki67 and height > 2cm (p=0.5)

By performing the t student test we did not find a statistically significant correlation between ki67 and tumor size (p=0.5).

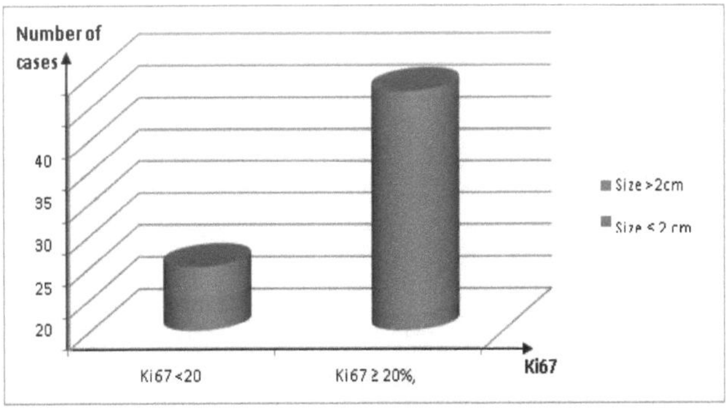

Figure 19 Ki67 index as a function of size

3.1.3. Correlation of Ki67 with histological type:

Invasive carcinoma was the most common histological type in patients with a Ki67 <20% (75.8% of cases) as well as in patients with Ki67≥ 20% (70% of cases). We did not find a statistically significant correlation between Ki67 and histological type (p=0.6). The distribution of Ki67 according to histological type is shown in Table II

Table II CorrelationKi67 and histological type:

Histological type	Ki67 <20	Ki67≥ 20%	p
Invasive carcinoma NOS	22	28	0,6
Lobular carcinoma	4	7	
Mixed carcinoma	3	3	
Carcinoma micropapillary	0	2	

3.1.4. Correlation of Ki67 with SBR grade: Figure 20

Among the 29 cases with Ki67<20%, seven had SBR Grade I (24.1% of cases), 18 had SBRI Grade II (62%), four had SBRI Grade II (13.9%).Among the 40 cases with Ki67 ≥ 20%, three had SBR Grade I (7.5% of cases), 15 had SBRI Grade II (37.5%), 21 had SBRI GradeII (52.5%).We found a statistically significant correlation between Ki67 and SBR grade (p=0.02)

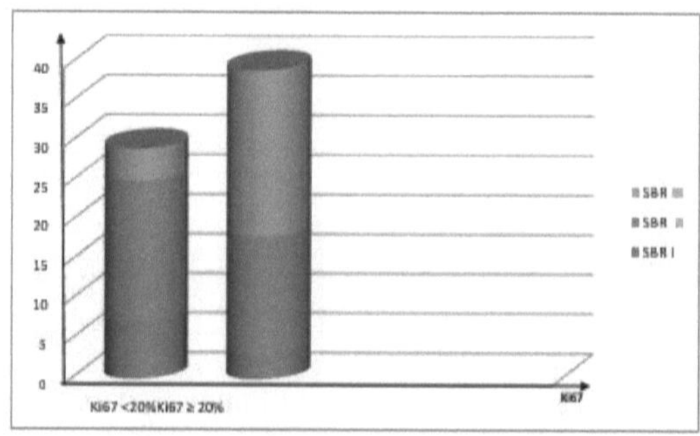

Figure 20 Ki67 index as a function of SBR grade

3.1.5. Correlation of Ki67 with architectural grade, nuclear grade and mitotic grade:

The correlation of Ki67 with architectural grade, nuclear grade and mitotic grade is represented in Table III.

Table III Ki67 and architectural grade, nuclear grade and mitotic grade

	Ki67 <20	Ki67≥ 20%	p
Architectural grade			0,05
Score 1	5	5	
Score 2	9	4	
Score 3	15	31	
Nuclear grade			0,6
Score 1	5	6	
Score 2	15	17	
Score 3	9	17	
Mitotic grade Score 1	19	11	0,04
Score 2	6	11	
Score 3	4	18	

3.1.6. Correlation of Ki67 with pT stage:

Among the 29 cases with a Ki67 <20

- six were classified as pT1 (20.7% of cases)
- 17 were classified as pT2 (58.6% of cases)
- Six were classified as pT3 (20.7% of cases)
- None were classified as pT4

Among the 40 cases with Ki67 ≥ 20%:

- Three were classified as pT1 (7.5% of cases)
- 29 were classified as pT2 (72.5% of cases)
- Five were classified as pT3 (12.5% of cases)
- Three were classified as pT4 (7.5% of cases)

We did not find a statistically significant correlation between Ki67 and stage pT (p=0,1)

3.1.7. Correlation of Ki67 with pN stage:

Among the 29 cases with Ki67 <20%:
- 11 were classified as pN0 (38% of cases).
- Nine were classified as pN1 (31% of cases).
- Five were classified as pN2 (17.2% of cases).
- Four were classified as pN3 (13.8% of cases).

Among the 40 cases with Ki67 ≥ 20%:

- 16 were classified pN0 (40% of cases)
- Eight were classified as pN1 (20% of cases)
- 11 were classified as pN2 (27.5% of cases)
- Five were classified as pN3 (15.9% of cases)

We did not find a statistically significant correlation between Ki67 and pN stage (p=0.6)

3.1.8. Correlation of Ki67 with vascular emboli:

Among the 29 cases with a Ki67 <20%, vascular emboli were present in seven cases (24.1% of cases).Among the 40 cases with Ki67 ≥ 20%, vascular emboli were present in 14 cases (35% of cases).

We did not find a statistically significant correlation between Ki67 and the presence of vascular emboli (p=0.4)

3.1.9. Correlation of Ki67 with perineural sheathing:

Among the 29 cases with Ki67 <20%, vascular emboli were present in nine cases (31% of cases).

Among the 40 cases with Ki67 ≥ 20%, vascular emboli were present in eight cases (20% of cases).

We did not find a statistically significant correlation between Ki67 and the presence of vascular emboli (p=0.3)

3.1.10. Correlation of Ki67 with ER, PR and HER 2 and molecular classification:

The correlation of Ki67 with ER, PR and HER 2 and the molecular classification is represented in Table IV

	Ki67 <20%	Ki67 ≥ 20%	P
Receivers with estrogen			0,03
< 10%	25	25	
	4	15	
Progesterone receptors			0,03
< 10%	24		
≥ 10%	5	23	
		17	
HER2			0,07
Not overexpressed	23	24	
Overexpressed	6	16	
Classification molecular			< 10-3
Luminal A	19	1	
Luminal B	7	26	
HER2	2	6	
Triple negative	1	7	

Table IV Ki67 as a function of estrogen receptor (ER), progesterone receptor (PR), HER2 and molecular classification

3.1.11. In total:

We found a statistically significant correlation between Ki67 and :

- SBR grade (p=0.02)

- architectural grade (p=0.05)

- mitotic grade (p=0.04)

- ERs (p=0.03)

- PR (p=0.03)

- molecular classification (p<10-3)

3.2. Multivariate analysis:

Multivariate analysis including SBR grade, architectural grade, mitotic grade, ER, PR, and molecular classification showed that molecular classification was the independent factor (p<10-3).

DISCUSSIONS

1. Key findings of the study:

Our study included 69 cases of CS collected over a five-year period from the first

January 2016 to December 31, 2021.

The average age of the patients was 53 years. The average tumor size was 35 mm.

The main histological type found was invasive carcinoma without other indication (NOS) (72.5% of cases).

The pT2 stage was the majority stage (66.7% of cases).

The tumor was SBR grade I in 14.5%, SBR II in 47.8% and SBR III in 37.7% of cases.

Luminal B molecular subtype was the most frequent representing 47.8% of cases, followed by Luminal A present in 29% of cases and HER2 subtypes in 11.6% of cases and triple negative in 11.6% of cases.

The ki67 index was $\geq 20\%$ in 58% of cases.

We found a statistically significant correlation between Ki67 and :

- SBR grade (p=0.02)
- architectural grade (p=0.05)
- mitotic grade (p=0.04)
- ERs (p=0.03)
- PR (p=0.03)
- molecular classification (p<10-3)

We found no statistically significant correlation between Ki67 and age (p=0.5), tumor size, histologic type (p=0.6), pT stage (p=0.1), pN stage(p=0.6), nuclear grade (p=0.6), vascular emboli (p=0.4), perineural engraftment (p=0.3), and HER2 status (p=0.07).

2. Epidemiological characteristics:

2.1. Impact:

SC is the most common cancer worldwide [1]. However, the incidence of SC varies considerably from country to country with a tendency for higher incidence rates in developed countries [12]. This could be explained by genetic factors but also by socioeconomic risk factors (obesity, sedentary lifestyle, parity, lack of breastfeeding, alcohol consumption, high-protein diet and high standard of living). The standardized incidence rate of CS according to geographic area is represented in Table V. The incidence of CS is 2-4 times lower in North Africa than in Western countries [13].

CS is the most frequent cancer in our country with a standardized incidence rate of 31.8/100000 inhabitants [1,14]. This rate is quite close to that of developing countries (30.7/100000 inhabitants) and North African countries [12].

Table V Standardized incidence rate of breast cancer by geographic area
[12,14].

Geographical area	Standardized incidence/100000 population
World	46.3
Australia	94.2
Europe	90.1
North America	84.8
North Africa	27.9
Central Asia	25.9
Tunisia	31.8
Developed countries	75.2
Developing countries	30.7

2.2. Age at diagnosis:

Age is one of the major non-modifiable risk factors for CS. However, age at diagnosis varies according to the geographical distribution of patients. The age of patients at diagnosis is younger in low- and middle-income countries (LMICs) than in high-income countries (HICs), with the average age of patients at diagnosis approximately 10 years younger in LMICs than in HICs [15]. This is partly due to the age distribution in developing countries, which favors a younger population compared to developed countries [13].

These carcinomas occurring at younger ages would tend to be more aggressive, with higher histological grades, more marked proliferation indexes and more vascular emboli [16].

In our series, the mean age of the patients at the time of diagnosis was 53 years. It was consistent with the values reported in other Tunisian series [17,18], (see Table VII). However, it was significantly lower than that reported in Western studies [19-21]. The comparison with worldwide series is reported in Table VI.

Table VI Age at diagnosis of CS according to series [4,19-25].

Authors	Country	Average age at diagnosis (in years)
Balekouzou et al	South Africa	45,8
Darré et al	Togo	46,3
Nishit et al	India	47,4
Al-Nuaimi et al	Iraq	50,4
Kanyılmaz et al.	Turkie	52
Our series	Tunisia	53
Nishimura et al	Japan	56,2
Hennings et al	Germany	57
Parker et al	United States	58
Al Jarrah et al	Great Britain	61

3. Anatomopathological characteristics:

3.1. Tumor size:

In our series, the mean tumor size was 35 mm. It was close to the average tumor size reported in Tunisian series [17,26], (see Table VII). However, the mean tumor size was significantly smaller in Western studies (20-22 mm) [4,27]. This reflects the fact that Tunisian patients consult rather late. This can be explained by the lack of awareness, access to screening and care facilities and the fact that mammography is not free. Hence the importance of establishing a national screening program for breast cancer in our country.

3.2. Histological type:

The most frequent histological type in our study was invasive carcinoma without other indication (NOS) (72.5% of cases). This is in line with the data from the Tunisian cancer registry of the northern region, which indicated that NOS represented 80.7% of all diagnosed SC [2]. It was also the predominant histological type in studies: Tunisian (Sahraoui et al: 77% of cases [24], Limam et al 72.5% [18]), Indian (Hungund et al 86% [28]), Afghan (Hashmi et al: 86.8%), Japanese (Nishimura et al: 83.1% of cases [4]) and German (Hennings et al (85.5%) [19].

3.3. Histological grade:

In our series SBR grade II was the most represented (47.8% of cases). This was in agreement with the results of Erić et al (48.5%), Hennings et al 53.4% and some Tunisian studies [18,29-31]. However, our results contrasted with those of a Tunisian study and an Iraqi study where SBR III grade tumors were the most frequent representing 41% and 46.4% of cases respectively [26,32]. This reflects the fact that SC tends to be more aggressive in underdeveloped countries.

3.4. Stage pT:

In our series, the most common tumor stage was pT2 (66% of cases). Similar results have been found in many Tunisian studies [17, 18, 30]. In our review of the literature, we found that pT1 stages were predominant in western series (49.9%-61.2%) [19,21], whereas pT3 and pT4 stages were predominant in sub-Saharan series [33-35]. This confirms the gap between developed and underdeveloped countries in the early diagnosis of SC and attests that SC is diagnosed much later in underdeveloped and developing countries than in developed countries. This is a further argument in favor of the benefits of systematic screening programs for the target population.

3.5. Molecular classification:

Luminal B subtype was the most frequent in our series (47.8% of cases). Similar results were found in the study by Berg et al [36]. However, our results were discordant with those of several Tunisian [26,37], African [22,35], Japanese [4,38] and Western [16,19] studies where the most frequent molecular subtype was Luminal A. The observed differences could be related to the fact that the distinction between Luminal A and B subtypes is partly made by the Ki67 index. The lack of reproducibility of this index and the use of different thresholds from one pathologist to another mean that some Luminal A tumors could have been classified as Luminal B and vice versa.

	Average age	Average tumor size	More frequent histological type	the	SBR grade more prevalent	the	Under type Molecular the most represented	StageT most represented	the	Most represented N stage
Our series	53	35	72.5		II (47.8%)		LuminalB (47.8%)	T2 (66.7%)		N0 (39.2%)
Limam et al	49.3	30	78.7%		II (43.4%)			T2 (42.6%)		N0 (64.1%)
Ben Gobrane et al	49.7	49	80.4%		II (53.3%)					
Missaoui et al	50.5				II (46.6%)			T2 (49.2%)		
Fourati et al	50.7	31			II (48.8%)		Luminal A (50.7%)			
Sahraoui et al	51		77%		III (41%)		Luminal A (64.1%)			
Belaid et al	50	35			II (51.5%)			T2 (44.7%)		N1 (31.9%)

3.6. Index Ki 67

3.6.1. Definition and History:

Ki 67 is a gene encoding a non-histone nuclear protein of 395 KD, described in 1983 by Gerdes from a monoclonal mouse immunization model by injection of Hodgkin's disease tumor cell nuclei [39].

The expression of Ki67, which varies according to the different phases of the cell cycle, is null in G0 phase, low in S, G1 and G2 phases and higher in with a peak in M [39,40].

A significant correlation was found between the rate of positive cells expressing Ki 67 and mitotic index in CS [40].

In addition, Ki 67 is one of 21 prospectively selected genes included in the Oncotype DX™ assay used to predict recurrence risk and chemotherapy efficacy in women with node-negative RE-positive breast cancer [41].

3.6.2. Method for determining Ki67:

Immunohistochemistry is the technique of choice to evaluate the Ki67 index. This index is expressed as a percentage ranging from 0% to 100%. This is the percentage of infiltrating tumor cells that are positively labeled in relation to the total tumor cells. The count must be done on at least 500 infiltrating tumor cells. Only nuclear labelling is taken into account, regardless of the intensity of the labelling (weak, moderate or intense).The two most commonly used methods for the determination of the Ki67 index are:

- The Hot Spot method: pathologists are mainly interested in Hot Spot fields (areas with the highest rate of Ki76-labeled tumor cells). The counting must be done, at high magnification (x400), on at least 3 Hot Spot fields. The Hot Spot fields present in the invasion front must be included in the count in a systematic way.

- The global method: The whole slide is analyzed at low magnification (x100). The counting is done at high magnification (x400) on at least three distinct fields, with different rates of Ki67 labeling. If a hot spot field is present, it must be included in the count [42].

To date, there is no real consensus on the method to be used. The 2019 WHO classification of CS does not specify which method to use. Several studies have compared these two methods. A multicenter study, conducted in 2019, involving 23 pathologists from 12 different countries had established that there was no statistically significant difference between these two methods [43].

3.6.3. Threshold values or "cut-offs" of the Ki67 index:

The threshold value of Ki67 is still a subject of dispute in the absence of a true consensus. It has evolved over time.In 2009, Cheang et al. had used the ki67 index in a study of 357 patients to separate luminal A and B tumor subtypes in a manner similar to that determined by the expression profile of 50 genes (PAM 50) [44]. In this study, the ki67 cut-off value was set at 13.25% to discriminate low-proliferating luminal A tumors from high-proliferating luminal B tumors. The 10-year survival of patients with luminal B tumors was 79%, whereas survival was 92% for luminal A tumors (p < 0.001). Taking into account the data of this study, the St. Gallen Consensus Conference in 2011 had retained the cutoff value of 14% to distinguish between luminal A and B tumors and decide the indication for adjuvant therapy [45].

In 2013, the experts at the St. Gallen conference, had proposed the cut-off value of 20% (Ki67 positive or high if ≥ 20%), while accepting local, laboratory-specific specificities that would choose a lower cut-off value to define a "positive" Ki67 [46]. They had based this on the fact that several studies had shown that the 20% Ki67 cutoff was a significant factor for overall survival in the Luminal B subtype.However, at the 2015 consensus meeting in St. Gallen, the minimum Ki67 value required for the definition of luminal subtype B, was for the majority of experts, between 20 and 29% [47]. Due to the persistence of intra- and inter-observer and laboratory variability, the expert panel had finally proposed that each laboratory should define and use its own Ki67 cut-off value offering the best inter-observer agreement between pathologists in that laboratory [47].

More recently, in 2019, the International Ki67 in Breast Cancer Working Group had ruled that a ki67<5% index was associated with a better prognosis and that a ki67>30% correlated with a poor prognosis and that chemotherapy could be proposed in this case [10].

A comparison between the different threshold values adopted in different studies is shown in Table VIII.

Table VIII Adopted cut-off values of Ki67 index according to studies [48-53]

Authors	Year of study	Numbers of patients in the study	Value included	threshold of the Ki67 index
Fasching et al	2011	552		13%
Petrelli et al	2015	64196		25%
Enrico et al	2018	506		20%
Wu et al	2019	7716		40%
Zhu et al	2020	1800		30%
Tian et al	2020	1008		15%

3.6.4. Inter-observer variability

Various studies had explored the reproducibility of the Ki67 index. E the results were discordant. Polley et al had established that intra-laboratory reproducibility was high (ICC =0.94; CI95% = 0.93 to 0.97). In contrast, inter-laboratory reproducibility was moderate (95% CI = 0.37 to 0.68). Another study reported a poor correlation in the evaluation of Ki67 by 6 pathologists from the same laboratory (ICC = 0.57).

3.6.5. Distribution according to ki67 :

The ki67 index was $\geq 20\%$ in 58% of the cases studied. This was consistent with the work of Madani et al (ki67 was $\geq 20\%$ in 55.4 cases) [31] and Nishimura et al (54.4%). However, this Ki67 was $\geq 20\%$ in less than 50% of cases studied in several series [25,38]. These discrepancies can be explained by the fact that, in the absence of a true consensus, different methods are used to evaluate the Ki67 index resulting in poor reproducibility and high inter-observer variability. Moreover, as the threshold values are not yet well codified, each team of pathologists opts for its own threshold value. This high interobserver variability and lack of reproducibility have limited the adoption of the Ki67 index in clinical practice [43]. Indeed, the assessment of Ki67 in a systematic way for all CS cases is not recommended in most population-based studies and meta-analyses [54]. The use of digitized methods could overcome these shortcomings.

3.6.6. Correlation of Ki67 index with histopronostic factors of CS:
a) Correlation of Ki67 with age:

We did not find a statistically significant correlation between Ki67 index and age. These results are consistent with the majority of studies [24,28,32,55,56]. However, two Japanese studies [4,38] had reported a statistically significant correlation between Ki67 index and age with p< 10-3. These differences between the series could be explained by the differences between the mean ages reported in each series and by the fact that different thresholds were used to evaluate the Ki67 index.

b) Correlation of Ki67 with height:

In our series, the Ki67 index was not correlated with tumor size. Similar results have been found in many studies [5,24,28]. In contrast, Ragab et al showed a statistically significant correlation between Ki67 index and tumor size (p=0.01) [55]. This correlation was also reported in the study of Nishimura et al (p<10-3) [4] and that of Sun p<0.05 [56]. The discordant results between the different studies can be explained by the use of different macroscopic management protocols of the surgical specimens as well as the high interobserver variability and lack of reproducibility of the Ki67 index.

c) Correlation of Ki67 with histological type:

Several studies agree that there is no statistically significant correlation between Ki67 index and histological type [16,28,32,55,56]. This was also found in our study (p=0.6).

d) Correlation of Ki67 with SBR grade:

We established that there was a statistically significant relationship between Ki67 and SBR grade (p=0.02). This agrees with the results of many studies Haroon et al (p=0.01) [5], Ushimado et al [38], Kanyılmaz et al (p<10-3) [25], Hungund et al (p=0.05) [28] and Erić (p=0.04) [16]. These results could be explained in part by the fact that mitotic grade is one component of SBR grade. As the prognosis of SC is directly correlated with the SBR stage [57], this would be a further argument for the prognostic role of Ki67 index in SC.

e) Correlation of Ki67 with pT stage

Our study had not revealed any correlation between Ki67 and pT stage. Similar results were reported by Ragab et al [55] and Haroon et al [5]. In contrast, Erić et al [16] and Ushimado et al [38] had found a correlation between high Ki67 and more advanced pT stage (p=0.001).

f) Correlation of Ki67 with pN stage:

In our series, a ki67 index≥ 20% was not associated with a higher risk of developing lymph node metastases. This agreed with the data reported by Ragab et al [55] who did not find a correlation between Ki67 and pN stage (p=0.3). Similarly, Nishit al had reached the same conclusions (p=0.8)

g) Correlation of Ki67 with ER and PR:

In our study, we found that the Ki67 index was inversely correlated with the levels of ER (p=0.03) and PR (p=0.03). A high Ki67 index was associated with low levels of ER and PR. These results are consistent with those of Japanese [4,38], Pakistani [5] and German [58] studies.

h) Correlation of Ki67 with HER 2

In our study, we found a correlation but not statistically significant (p=0.07) between the Ki67 index and HER2 status. This result could be biased by the fact that we did not have a molecular biology technique to better explore the HER2 score and verify if it is really an overexpressed HER2. Several studies had established a correlation between Ki67 index and HER2 status [4,27,28].

i) Correlation of Ki67 with molecular stage:

A strong correlation between Ki67 index and molecular classification was demonstrated by our study(p<10-3). Similar results have been reported by several studies [25]

Breast cancer (BC) is a major public health problem in Tunisia. It is the most common cancer and the second most common cause of death by cancer in our country. Breast cancer, being a rather heterogeneous and complex disease, its prognosis depends on several interrelated factors. The most commonly recognized histopronostic factors of SC were histological type, tumor size, tumor grade, vascular emboli and lymph node involvement. The continuous search for new histopronostic factors for patients with SC is imperative in view of its increasing incidence and mortality worldwide and in Tunisia.

During the last twenty years, there has been a growing interest in the biology of SC and molecular classification has become a gold standard and a necessity for most teams. Indeed, the American Association of Clinical Oncology (ASCO) recommends the evaluation of estrogen and progesterone receptor levels as well as the HER2 score in a systematic way for all cases of SC.

The ki67 index is the most commonly used proliferation marker. Although there is no real consensus on the method of determination and the cut-off values to be adopted, several studies have shown that it is a major prognostic factor in SC. A low Ki67 is correlated with a good response to chemotherapy, a better survival and a low risk of recurrence.Although the prognostic value of the Ki67 index has been widely studied, few studies had investigated the correlation of the Ki67 index with conventional prognostic factors of CS.

We conducted a retrospective descriptive study of CS cases diagnosed in the Department of Pathological Anatomy and Cytology of Habib Thameur Hospital over a period of five years.Our objectives were to study the clinico-pathological characteristics of CS in a university hospital in northern Tunisia and to evaluate the correlation of the Ki67 index with the main prognostic factors of CS.To our knowledge, this is the first study to evaluate the correlation of the Ki67 index with the main prognostic factors of CS conducted in Tunisia and North

Africa.We collected 69 cases. The average age of the patients was 53 years. The tumor size average was 35mm. The main histological type found was invasive carcinoma without other indication (NOS) (72.5% of cases). The pT2 stage was the majority stage (66.7% of cases).The tumor was SBR grade I in 14.5%, SBR II in 47.8% and SBR III in 37.7% of cases.Luminal B molecular subtype was the most frequent representing 47.8% of cases, followed by Luminal A present in 29% of cases and HER2 subtypes in 11.6% of cases and triple negative in 11.6% of cases. The ki67 index was $\geq$ 20% in 58% of cases.We found a statistically significant correlation between Ki67 and SBR grade (p=0.02), architectural grade (p=0.05), mitotic grade (p=0.04), ERs (p=0.03), PRs (p=0.03) and molecular classification (p<10-3).We found no statistically significant correlation between Ki67 and age (p=0.5), tumor size, histologic type (p=0.6), pT stage (p=0.1), pN stage(p=0.6), nuclear grade (p=0.6), vascular emboli (p=0.4), perineural engraftment (p=0.3), and HER2 status (p=0.07). Our study established that the Ki67 index was correlated with many conventional histopronostic factors of CS. This is a further argument in favor of the prognostic role of Ki67 index in CS and encourages its systematic evaluation and transcription on all pathological reports of CS. Additional studies with larger numbers would be necessary to confirm our results. A consensus unifying the methods of determination of the Ki67 index and the threshold values to be adopted would make it possible to overcome the insufficiencies of this index, to limit the difficulties encountered by pathologists during its evaluation and to facilitate its use in current clinical practice.

REFERENCES

1.Sung H, Ferlay J, Siegel RL, Laversanne M, Soerjomataram I, Jemal A, et al. Global Cancer Statistics 2020: GLOBOCAN Estimates of Incidence and Mortality Worldwide for 36 Cancers in 185 Countries. CA Cancer J Clin. 2021 May;71(3):209-49.

2.North Tunisia Cancer Registry.

3.K D, A S, O S, H BR. Cancer mortality among reproductive age women in Tunisia. Tunis Med [Internet]. 2016 Jan [cited 2022 Apr 17];94(1). Available from: https://pubmed.ncbi.nlm.nih.gov/27525600/

4.Nishimura R, Osako T, Okumura Y, Hayashi M, Toyozumi Y, Arima N. Ki67 as a prognostic marker according to breast cancer subtype and a predictor of recurrence time in primary breast cancer. Exp Ther Med. 2010;1(5):747-54.

5.Haroon S, Hashmi AA, Khurshid A, Kanpurwala MA, Mujtuba S, Malik B, et al. Ki67 Index in Breast Cancer: Correlation with Other Prognostic Markers and Potential in Pakistani Patients. Asian Pac J Cancer Prev. 2013 Jul 30;14(7):4353-8.

6.Hungund BR, Malur PR, Godhi AS. Ki67 Expression and Its Association with Conventional Prognostic Markers in Breast Carcinoma. Int J Health Sci Res. 2019;9(1):215-22.

7.de Azambuja E, Cardoso F, de Castro G, Colozza M, Mano MS, Durbecq V, et al. Ki67 as prognostic marker in early breast cancer: a meta-analysis of published studies involving 12 155 patients. Br J Cancer. 2007 May;96(10):1504-13.

8.Émile JF, Leteurtre E, Guyétant S. General pathology: thematic teaching, tissue, cellular and molecular biopathology. 3rd ed. Issy-les-Moulineaux:

Elsevier Masson; 2021. (DFGSM 2- 3 medicine).

9.PREPARATION OF A HISTOLOGICAL BLADE [Internet]. University of Oran - Faculty of Medicine; 2019. Available from: https://facmed-univ-oran.dz/resources/product_files/product_file_2500.pdf

10. Nielsen TO, Leung SCY, Rimm DL, Dodson A, Acs B, Badve S, et al. Assessment of Ki67 in Breast Cancer: Updated Recommendations From the International Ki67 in Breast Cancer Working Group. JNCI J Natl Cancer Inst. 2021 Jul 1;113(7):808-19.

11. F. Penault-Llorca, B. Bayol, N. Radosevic-Robin N 2017. Ki67 assessment in breast cancer: news Correspondences in Onco-Theranostics - Vol. VI - n° 1 - January-February-March 2017.

12. Huang J, Chan PS, Lok V, Chen X, Ding H, Jin Y, et al. Global incidence and mortality of breast cancer: a trend analysis. Aging. 2021 Feb 28;13(4):5748-803.

13. Corbex M, Bouzbid S, Boffetta P. Features of breast cancer in developing countries, examples from North-Africa. Eur J Cancer. 2014 Jul;50(10):1808-18.

14. Ministry of Health, Republic of Tunisia. PLAN FOR THE FIGHT AGAINST CANCER IN TUNISIA 2015-2019.

15. Bidoli E, Virdone S, Hamdi-Cherif M, Toffolutti F, Taborelli M, Panato C, et al. Worldwide Age at Onset of Female Breast Cancer: A 25-Year Population-Based Cancer Registry Study. Sci Rep. 2019 Dec;9(1):14111.

16. Erić I. Breast Cancer in Young Women: Pathologic and Immunohistochemical Features. Acta Clin Croat [Internet]. 2018 [cited 2022 May 1]; Available from: https://hrcak.srce.hr/index.php?show=clanak&id_clanak_jezik=315417

17. Belaid I, Fatma LB, Ezzairi F, Hochlaf M, Chabchoub I, Gharbi O, et al. Trends and current challenges of breast cancer in Tunisia: a retrospective study of 1262 cases with survival analysis. Breast J. 2018 Sep;24(5):846-8.

18. Limam M, Ajmi T, Zedini C, Khelifi A, Mellouli M, Ghardallou ME, et al. Study of breast cancer treatment waiting times in Sousse, Tunisia. Public Health (Bucur). 2016 Aug 12;28(3):331-40.

19. Hennigs A, Riedel F, Gondos A, Sinn P, Schirmacher P, Marmé F, et al. Prognosis of breast cancer molecular subtypes in routine clinical care: A large prospective cohort study. BMC Cancer. 2016 Dec;16(1):734.

20. Parker JS, Mullins M, Cheang MCU, Leung S, Voduc D, Vickery T, et al. Supervised Risk Predictor of Breast Cancer Based on Intrinsic Subtypes. J Clin Oncol. 2009 Mar 10;27(8):1160-7.

21. Aljarrah A, Miller WR. Trends in the distribution of breast cancer over time in the southeast of Scotland and review of the literature. Ecancermedicalscience. 2014;8:427.

22. Balekouzou A, Yin P, Pamatika CM, Bishwajit G, Nambei SW, Djeintote M, et al. Epidemiology of breast cancer: retrospective study in the Central African Republic. BMC Public Health. 2016 Dec;16(1):1230.

23. Darre T, Amégbor K, Sonhaye L, Kouyate M, Aboubaraki A, N'timo2 B, et al. Histo-epidemiological profile of breast cancer a report of 450 cases observed in the University Teaching Hospital of Lome. Médecine Afr Noire. 2013 Jan 1;2.

24. . N, Nigam JS, Kumar T, Bharti S, . S, Sinha R, et al. Association of Ki67 With Clinicopathological Factors in Breast Cancer. Cureus [Internet]. 2021 Jun 13 [cited 2022 Apr 28]; Available from: https://www.cureus.com/articles/61636-association-of-Ki67-with-clinicopathological-factors-in- breast-cancer

25. Department of Radiation Oncology, Necmettin Erbakan University, Meram School of Medicine, Konya, Turkey, Kanyilmaz G, Benli Yavuz B, Department of Radiation Oncology, Necmettin Erbakan University, Meram School of Medicine, Konya, Turkey, Aktan M, Department of Radiation Oncology, Necmettin Erbakan University, Meram School of Medicine, Konya, Turkey, et al. Prognostic Importance of Ki67 in Breast Cancer and Its Relationship with Other Prognostic Factors. Eur J Breast Health. 2019 Oct 1;15(4):256-61.

26. Sahraoui G, Khanchel F, Chelbi E. Anatomopathological profile of breast cancer in the Tunisian cap bon. Pan Afr Med J [Internet]. 2017 [cited 2022 Apr 29];26. Available from: http://www.panafrican-med-journal.com/content/article/26/11/full/

27. Alco G, Bozdogan A, Selamoglu D, Pilanci KN, Tuzlali S, Ordu C, et al. Clinical and histopathological factors associated with Ki67 expression in breast cancer patients. Oncol Lett. 2015 Mar;9(3):1046- 54.

28. Hungund B, Malur P, Godhi A, Tyagi N, Joshi A. Ki67 Expression and Its Association with Conventional Prognostic Markers in Breast Carcinoma. 2019 Jan 1;215.

29. Ben Gobrane, H., Fakhfakh, R., Rahal, K., Ben Ayed, F., Maalej, M. et al (2007). [Breast cancer prognosis in Salah Azaiez Institute of Cancer, Tunis]. EMHJ - Eastern Mediterranean Health Journal, 13 (2), 309-318, 2007.

30. Missaoui N, Jaidene L, Abdelkrim SB, Abdelkader AB, Beizig N, Yaacoub LB, et al. Breast cancer in Tunisia: clinical and pathological findings. Asian Pac J Cancer Prev APJCP. 2011;12(1):169-72.

31. Madani SH, Payandeh M, Sadeghi M, Motamed H, Sadeghi E. The correlation between Ki67 with other prognostic factors in breast cancer: A study in Iranian patients. Indian J Med Paediatr Oncol. 2016 Apr;37(02):95-9.

32. Al-Nuaimi H, Hamdi E, Mohammed B. Ki67 Expression in Breast Cancer, Its Correlation with ER, PR and Other Prognostic Factors in Nineveh Province. Ann Coll Med Mosul. 2020 Jun 1;42(1):1-10.

33. Togo A, Traoré A, Traoré C, Dembélé BT, Kanté L, Diakité I, et al. Breast cancer in two hospitals in Bamako, Mali: diagnostic and therapeutic aspects. J Afr Cancer Afr J Cancer. 2010 May;2(2):88-91.

34. Ranaivomanana M, Emile Hasiniatsy NR, Rakotomahenina H, Rafaramino F. Epidemioclinical aspects of breast cancers in the oncology department of Fianarantsoa, Madagascar from 2011 to 2018. Pan Afr Med J [Internet]. 2021 [cited 2022 May 1];38. Available from: https://www.panafrican- med-journal.com/content/article/38/264/full

35. Elgaili EM, Abuidris DO, Rahman M, Michalek AM, Mohammed SI. Breast cancer burden in central Sudan. Int J Womens Health. 2010 Aug 9;2:77-82.

36. van den Berg EJ, Duarte R, Dickens C, Joffe M, Mohanlal R. Ki67 Immunohistochemistry Quantification in Breast Carcinoma: A Comparison of Visual Estimation, Counting, and ImmunoRatio. Appl Immunohistochem Mol Morphol AIMM. 2021 Feb 1;29(2):105-11.

37. Fourati A, Boussen H, El May MV, Goucha A, Dabbabi B, Gamoudi A, et al. Descriptive analysis of molecular subtypes in Tunisian breast cancer: Biomarkers and breast cancer. Asia Pac J Clin Oncol. 2014 Jun;10(2):e69-74.

38. Ushimado K, Kobayashi N, Hikichi M, Tsukamoto T, Urano M, Utsumi T. Inverse correlation between Ki67 expression as a continuous variable and outcomes in luminal HER2-negative breast cancer. Fujita Med J. 2019;5(3):728.

39. Gerdes J, Li L, Schlueter C, Duchrow M, Wohlenberg C, Gerlach C, et al. Immunobiochemical and molecular biologic characterization of the cell proliferation-associated nuclear antigen that is defined by monoclonal antibody Ki67. Am J Pathol. 1991 Apr;138(4):867-73.

40. El Benna H, Zribi A, Laabidi S, Haddaoui A, Mlika M, Skhiri H, et al. Ki67: role in diagnosis, prognosis and follow-up after treatment of breast cancers. Tunis Med. 2015 Dec;93(12):737-41.

41. Paik S, Tang G, Shak S, Kim C, Baker J, Kim W, et al. Gene Expression and Benefit of Chemotherapy in Women With Node-Negative, Estrogen Receptor-Positive Breast Cancer. J Clin Oncol. 2006 Aug 10;24(23):3726-34.

42. Shui R, Yu B, Bi R, Yang F, Yang W. An Interobserver Reproducibility Analysis of Ki67 Visual Assessment in Breast Cancer. Schmitt F, editor. PLOS ONE. 2015 May 1;10(5):e0125131.

43. Leung SCY, Nielsen TO, Zabaglo LA, Arun I, Badve SS, Bane AL, et al. Analytical validation of a standardized scoring protocol for Ki67 immunohistochemistry on breast cancer excision whole sections: an international multicentre collaboration. Histopathology. 2019 Aug;75(2):225-35.

44. Cheang MCU, Chia SK, Voduc D, Gao D, Leung S, Snider J, et al. Ki67 Index, HER2 Status, and Prognosis of Patients With Luminal B Breast Cancer. JNCI J Natl Cancer Inst. 2009 May 20;101(10):736-50.

45. Goldhirsch A, Wood WC, Coates AS, Gelber RD, Thürlimann B, Senn HJ. Strategies for subtypes- dealing with the diversity of breast cancer: highlights of the St Gallen International Expert Consensus on the Primary Therapy of Early Breast Cancer 2011. Ann Oncol. 2011 Aug;22(8):1736- 47.

46. Goldhirsch A, Winer EP, Coates AS, Gelber RD, Piccart-Gebhart M, Thürlimann B, et al. Personalizing the treatment of women with early breast cancer: highlights of the St Gallen International Expert Consensus on the Primary Therapy of Early Breast Cancer 2013. Ann Oncol. 2013 Sep;24(9):2206-23.

47. Coates AS, Winer EP, Goldhirsch A, Gelber RD, Gnant M, Piccart-Gebhart M, et al. Tailoring therapies-improving the management of early breast cancer:

St Gallen International Expert Consensus on the Primary Therapy of Early Breast Cancer 2015. Ann Oncol. 2015 Aug;26(8):1533- 46.

48. Fasching PA, Heusinger K, Haeberle L, Niklos M, Hein A, Bayer CM, et al. Ki67, chemotherapy response, and prognosis in breast cancer patients receiving neoadjuvant treatment. BMC Cancer. 2011 Dec;11(1):486.

49. Petrelli F, Viale G, Cabiddu M, Barni S. Prognostic value of different cut-off levels of Ki67 in breast cancer: a systematic review and meta-analysis of 64,196 patients. Breast Cancer Res Treat. 2015 Oct;153(3):477-91.

50. Enrico DH, Hannois AR, Bravo I. Evaluation of the best cut-off point for Ki67 and progesterone receptor as a prognostic factor in hormone receptor-positive (HR+) breast cancer. J Clin Oncol. 2018 May 20;36(15_suppl):e12549-e12549.

51. Wu Q, Ma G, Deng Y, Luo W, Zhao Y, Li W, et al. Prognostic Value of Ki67 in Patients With Resected Triple-Negative Breast Cancer: A Meta-Analysis. Front Oncol [Internet]. 2019 [cited 2022 Apr 24];9. Available from: https://www.frontiersin.org/article/10.3389/fonc.2019.01068

52. Zhu X, Chen L, Huang B, Wang Y, Ji L, Wu J, et al. The prognostic and predictive potential of Ki67 in triple-negative breast cancer. Sci Rep. 2020 Dec;10(1):225.

53. Tian C, Fu L, Wei J, Yin P, Zhang H. Ki67 versus MammaPrint/BluePrint for assessing luminal type breast cancer. J Clin Oncol. 2020 May 20;38(15_suppl):e13673-e13673.

54. Pathmanathan N, Balleine RL. Ki67 and proliferation in breast cancer. J Clin Pathol. 2013 Jun;66(6):512-6.

55. Ragab HM, Samy N, Afify M, El Maksoud NA, Shaaban HM. Assessment of Ki67 as a potential biomarker in patients with breast cancer. J Genet Eng

Biotechnol. 2018 Dec;16(2):479-84.

56. Sun GS, Wang S, Wang Y. Expressions of Topo IIα and Ki67 in breast cancer and its clinicopathologic features and prognosis: Breast cancer, its clinicopathologic features & prognosis. Pak J Med Sci [Internet].2019 May2 [cited 2022 May 1];35(3). Available from: http://www.pjms.org.pk/index.php/pjms/article/view/81

57. Goldblum JR, Lamps LW, McKenney JK, Myers JL, Ackerman LV, Rosai J, editors. Rosai and Ackerman's surgical pathology. Eleventh edition. Philadelphia, PA: Elsevier; 2018. 2 p.

58. Inwald EC, Klinkhammer-Schalke M, Hofstädter F, Zeman F, Koller M, Gerstenhauer M, et al. Ki67 is a prognostic parameter in breast cancer patients: results of a large population-based cohort of a cancer registry. Breast Cancer Res Treat. 2013 Jun;139(2):539-52.

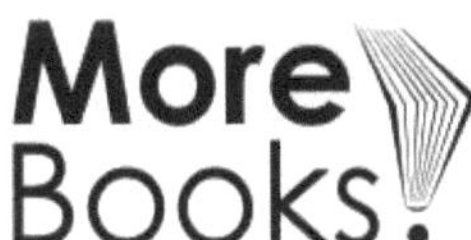

More
Books!

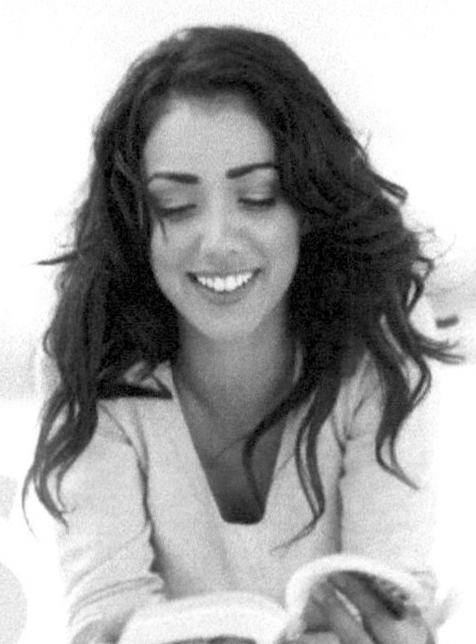

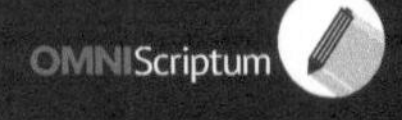

OMNIScriptum

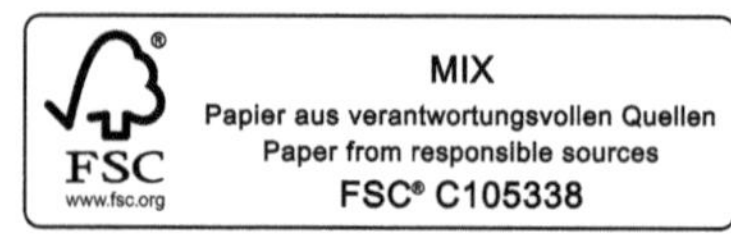

Printed by Books on Demand GmbH, Norderstedt / Germany